My Plant-Based Diet Cooking Guide

Creative and Easy Plant-Based Recipes

Luke Gorman

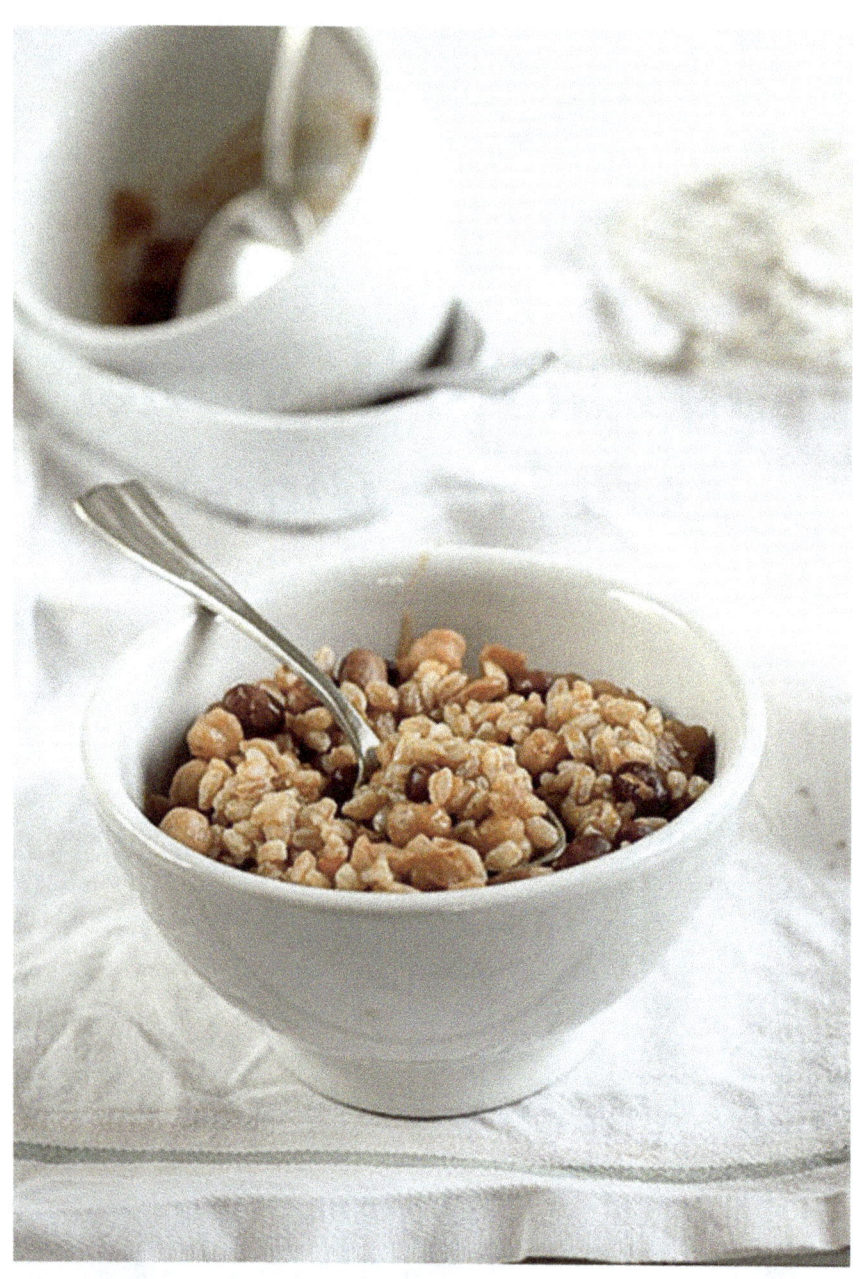

© Copyright 2021 - All rights reserved.

The content contained within this book may not be reproduced, duplicated or transmitted without direct written permission from the author or the publisher.
Under no circumstances will any blame or legal responsibility be held against the publisher, or author, for any damages, reparation, or monetary loss due to the information contained within this book. Either directly or indirectly.

Legal Notice:
This book is copyright protected. This book is only for personal use. You cannot amend, distribute, sell, use, quote or paraphrase any part, or the content within this book, without the consent of the author or publisher.

Disclaimer Notice:
Please note the information contained within this document is for educational and entertainment purposes only. All effort has been executed to present accurate, up to date, and reliable, complete information. No warranties of any kind are declared or implied. Readers acknowledge that the author is not engaging in the rendering of legal, financial, medical or professional advice. The content within this book has been derived from various sources. Please consult a licensed professional before attempting any techniques outlined in this book.
By reading this document, the reader agrees that under no circumstances is the author responsible for any losses, direct or indirect, which are incurred as a result of the use of information contained within this document, including, but not limited to, — errors, omissions, or inaccuracies.

TABLE OF CONTENTS

INTRODUCTION 7

CURRIED LENTIL SOUP 9

SIMPLE BLACK BEAN SOUP 11

SLOW COOKED SPLIT PEA SOUP 13

SLOW COOKER TUSCAN-STYLE SOUP 15

VITAMIN C-STOCKED BARLEY SOUP 17

GLAZED BEETS 19

EASY PEPPERS SIDE DISH 20

TOMATOES AND BASIL MIX 22

RED POTATOES AND GREEN BEANS 23

GOLD POTATOES AND BELL PEPPER MIX 24

EGGPLANT SALAD 26

SAVORY SPANISH RICE 28

TASTIEST BARBECUED TOFU AND VEGETABLES 30

SUPER TASTY VEGETARIAN CHILI 33

COMFORTING CHICKPEA TAGINE 35

FALAFEL 37

LEBANESE BEAN SALAD 40

LENTIL SOUP 42

QUINOA AND BLACK BEANS 44

STUFFED PEPPERS 46

VEGETABLE BARLEY SOUP 49

ASPARAGUS RICE PILAF 51

QUINOA AND BLACK BEAN CHILI 53

QUINOA WITH CHICKPEAS AND TOMATOES 55

ZUCCHINI RISOTTO 57

TOMATO BARLEY SOUP 59

LEMONY QUINOA 61

BROWN RICE, BROCCOLI, AND WALNUT 62

BROCCOLI AND RICE STIR FRY 64

COCONUT RICE 65

BROWN RICE PILAF 66

VEGAN CURRIED RICE 68

COCONUT CURRY LENTILS 71

CHARD WRAPS WITH MILLET 73

RICE STUFFED JALAPEÑOS 74

LENTIL AND WILD RICE SOUP 76

BLACK BEANS AND CAULIFLOWER RICE 78

BLACK BEAN AND QUINOA SALAD 80

COCONUT CHICKPEA CURRY 81

ZOODLES WITH WHITE BEANS 83

PASTA WITH KIDNEY BEAN SAUCE 85

CHICKPEA SHAKSHUKA 87

AVOCADO BURRITO BOWL.. 89

SWEET POTATO AND BEAN BURGERS 91

BURRITO-STUFFED SWEET POTATOES 93

SWEET POTATO, KALE AND CHICKPEA SOUP..................... 96

PESTO WITH SQUASH RIBBONS AND FETTUCCINE 98

THAI RED CURRY WITH VEGETABLES................................. 100

THAI GREEN CURRY WITH SPRING VEGETABLES 102

ZUCCHANOUSH.. 104

Introduction

A plant-based eating routine backing and upgrades the entirety of this. For what reason should most of what we eat originate from the beginning?

Eating more plants is the first nourishing convention known to man to counteract and even turn around the ceaseless diseases that assault our general public.

Plants and vegetables are brimming with large scale and micronutrients that give our bodies all that we require for a sound and productive life. By eating, at any rate, two suppers stuffed with veggies consistently, and nibbling on foods grown from the ground in the middle of, the nature of your wellbeing and at last your life will improve.

The most widely recognized wellbeing worries that individuals have can be reduced by this one straightforward advance.

Things like weight, inadequate rest, awful skin, quickened maturing, irritation, physical torment, and absence of vitality would all be able to be decidedly influenced by expanding the admission of plants and characteristic nourishments.

If you're reading this book, then you're probably on a journey to get healthy because you know good health and nutrition go hand in hand.

Maybe you're looking at the plant-based diet as a solution to those love handles.

Whatever the case may be, the standard American diet millions of people eat daily is not the best way to fuel your body.

If you ask me, any other diet will already be a significant improvement. Since what you eat fuels your body, you can imagine that eating junk will make you feel just that—like junk.

I've followed the standard American diet for several years: my plate was loaded with high-fat and carbohydrate-rich foods. I know this doesn't sound like a horrible way to eat, but keep in mind that most Americans don't focus on eating healthy fats and complex carbs—we live on processed foods.

The consequences of eating foods filled with trans fats, preservatives, and mountains of sugar are fatigue, reduced mental focus, mood swings, and weight gain. To top it off, there's the issue of opening yourself up to certain diseases—some life-threatening—when you neglect paying attention to what you eat .

Curried Lentil Soup

Preparation time: 5 minutes

Cooking time: 30 minutes

Servings: 5-6

Ingredients:

- 1 cup dried lentils
- 1 large onion, finely cut
- 1 celery rib, chopped
- 1 large carrot, chopped
- 3 garlic cloves, chopped
- 1 can tomatoes, undrained
- 3 cups vegetable broth
- 1 tbsp curry powder
- 1/2 tsp ground ginger

Directions:

1. Combine all ingredients in slow cooker.
2. Cover and cook on low for 5-6 hours.
3. Blend soup to desired consistency, adding additional hot water to thin, if desired.

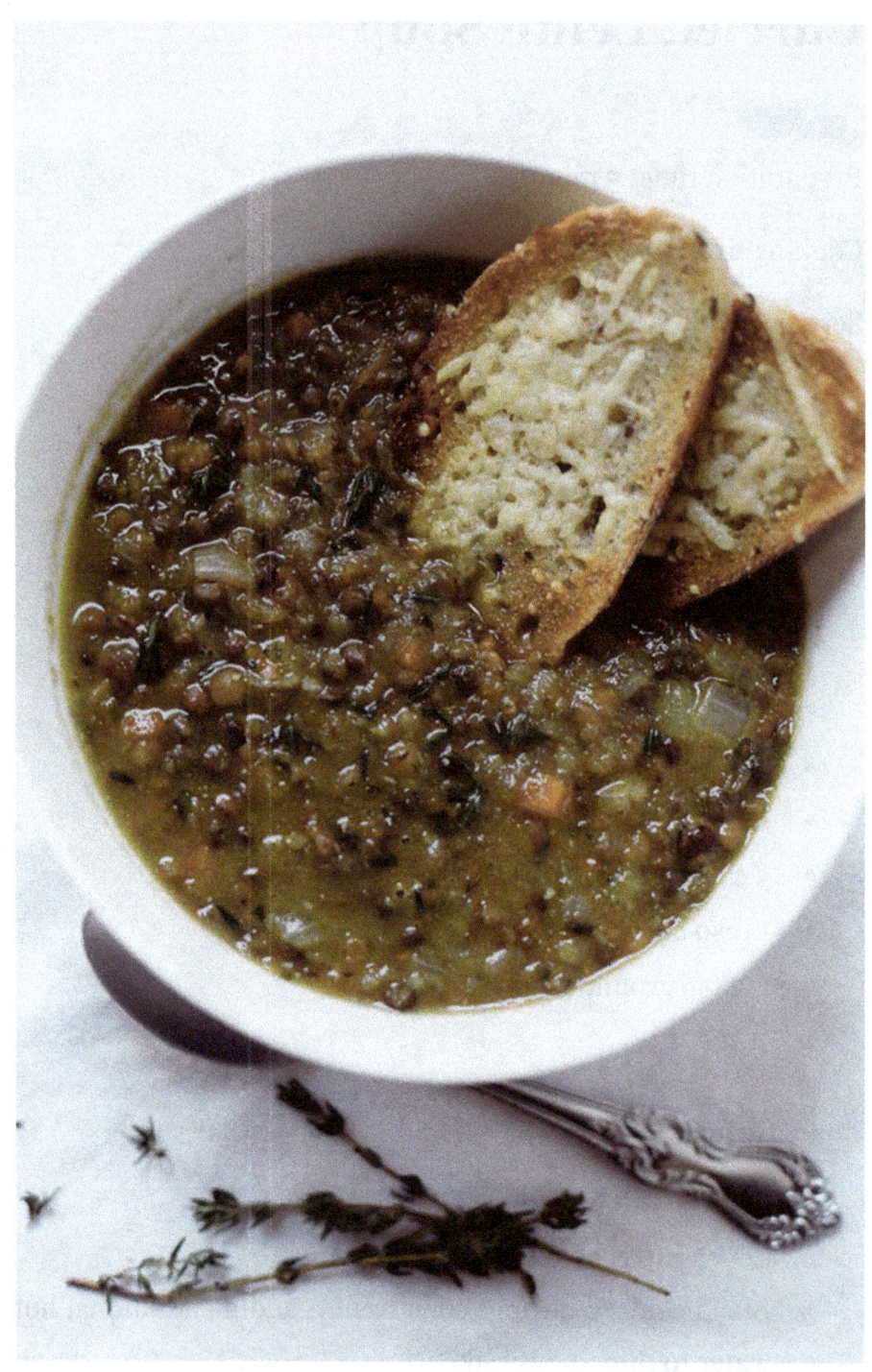

Simple Black Bean Soup

Preparation time: 5 minutes

Cooking time: 50 minutes

Servings: 5-6

Ingredients:

- 1 cup dried black beans
- 5 cups vegetable broth
- 1 large onion, chopped
- 1 red pepper, chopped
- 1 tsp sweet paprika
- 1 tbsp dried mint
- 2 bay leaves
- 1 Serrano chili, finely chopped
- 1 tsp salt
- 4 tbsp fresh lime juice
- 1/2 cup chopped fresh cilantro
- 1 cup vegan cream, to serve

Directions:

1. Wash the beans and soak them in enough water overnight.
2. In a slow cooker, combine the beans and all other ingredients except for the lime juice and cilantro.
3. Cover and cook on low for 7-8 hours.
4. Add salt, lime juice and fresh cilantro.
5. Serve with a dollop of vegan cream.

Slow Cooked Split Pea Soup

Preparation time: 5 minutes

Cooking time: 50 minutes

Servings: 5-6

Ingredients:

- 1 lb dried green split peas, rinsed and drained
- 2 potatoes, peeled and diced
- 1 small onion, chopped
- 1 celery rib, chopped
- 1 carrot, chopped
- 2 garlic cloves, chopped
- 1 bay leaf
- 1 tsp black pepper
- 1/2 tsp salt
- 6 cups water

Directions:

1. Combine all ingredients in slow cooker.
2. Cover and cook on low for 5-6 hours.
3. Discard bay leaf.

4. Blend soup to desired consistency, adding additional hot water to thin, if desired.
5. Serve with garlic or herb bread.

Slow Cooker Tuscan-style Soup

Preparation time: 5 minutes

Cooking time: 20 minutes

Servings: 5-6

Ingredients:

- 1 lb potatoes, peeled and cubed
- 1 small onion, chopped
- 1 can mixed beans, drained
- 1 carrot, chopped
- 2 garlic cloves, chopped
- 4 cups vegetable broth
- 1 cups chopped kale
- 3 tbsp olive oil
- 1 bay leaf salt and pepper, to taste
- Grated vegan cheese, to serve

Directions:

1. Heat oil in a skillet over medium heat and sauté the onion, carrot and garlic, stirring, for 2-3 minutes or until soft.

2. Combine all ingredients except the kale into the slow cooker.
3. Season with salt and pepper to taste.
4. Cook on high for 4 hours or low for 6-7 hours.
5. Add in kale about 30 minutes before soup is finished cooking.
6. Serve sprinkled with vegan cheese.

Vitamin C-Stocked Barley Soup

Preparation time: 5 minutes

Cooking time: 60 minutes 10 cups.

Ingredients:

- 2 diced onions
- 1 tbsp. olive oil
- 4 minced garlic cloves
- 4 diced green onions
- 2 diced zucchinis
- 1 diced yellow pepper
- 3 diced carrots
- 5 cups vegetable broth
- 20 ounces diced tomatoes
- ½ cup buckwheat groats
- 1/3 cup pearled barley
- 2 tbsp. lemon juice
- 3 tbsp. parsley
- salt and pepper to taste

Directions:

1. Begin by heating the onion, the garlic, and the olive oil in the bottom of a large soup pot.
2. Heat them for eight minutes.
3. Next, add the spices and cook for an additional two minutes.
4. Add the rest of the vegetables, and cook them for five more minutes.
5. Next, add the broth, the diced tomatoes, the buckwheat, and the barley.
6. Allow the soup to simmer for twenty minutes.
7. Make sure to stir it every few moments.
8. Next, add the lemon juice and the rest of the spices you desire.
9. Cook the mixture for a few more minutes, stirring occasionally.
10. Then, serve warm, and enjoy!

Glazed Beets

Preparation Time: 10 minutes

Cooking Time: 50 minutes

Servings:

Ingredients

- 3 pounds beetroots, peeled and cut into medium chunks
- 4 tablespoons maple syrup
- 1 tablespoon olive oil

Directions:

1. Rub beets with the oil, add maple syrup, toss, introduce in your Air Fryer and cook at 350 ° F for 40 minutes.
2. Divide between plates and serve as a side dish.

Easy Peppers Side Dish

Preparation Time: 10 minutes

Cooking Time: 25 minutes

Servings: 1

Ingredients

- 12 colored bell peppers, seedless and sliced
- 1 tablespoon olive oil
- 1 yellow onion, sliced
- ½ teaspoon smoked paprika
- Salt and black pepper to the taste

Directions:

1. Put the oil in a pan that fits your Air Fryer, add bell peppers, paprika and onion, toss, introduce the pan in your Air Fryer and cook at 320 ° F for 25 minutes.
2. Season with salt and pepper to the taste, divide between plates and serve as a side dish.

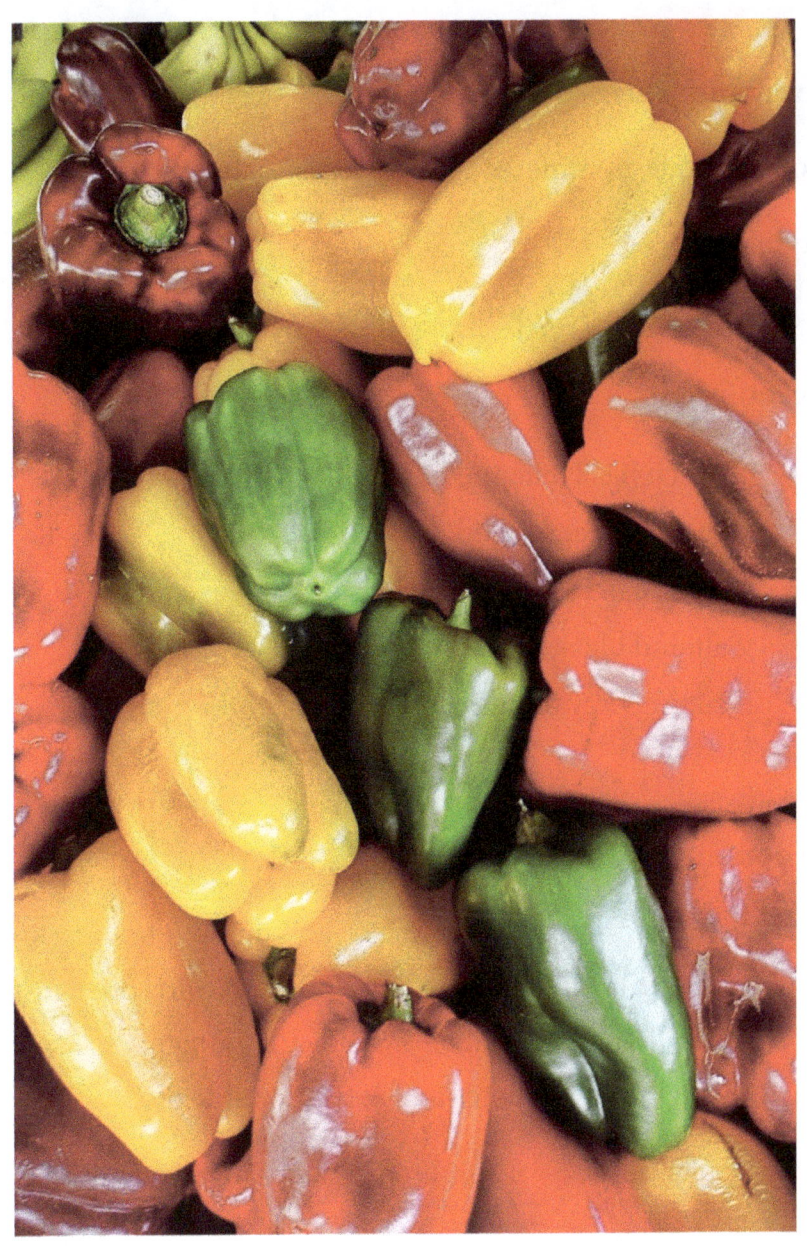

Tomatoes And Basil Mix

Preparation Time: 10 minutes

Cooking Time: 14 minutes

Servings:

Ingredients

- 1 bunch basil, chopped
- 3 garlic clove, minced
- A drizzle of olive oil
- Salt and black pepper to the taste
- 2 cups cherry tomatoes, halved

Directions:

1. In a pan that fits your Air Fryer, combine tomatoes with garlic, salt, pepper, basil and oil, toss, introduce in your Air Fryer and cook at 320 ° F for 12 minutes.
2. Divide between plates and serve as a side dish.

Red Potatoes And Green Beans

Preparation Time: 10 minutes

Cooking Time: 15 minutes

Servings:

Ingredients

- 1 pound red potatoes, cut into wedges
- 1 pound green beans
- 2 garlic cloves, minced
- 2 tablespoons olive oil
- Salt and black pepper to the taste
- ½ teaspoon oregano, dried

Directions:

1. In a pan that fits your Air Fryer, combine potatoes with green beans, garlic, oil, salt, pepper and oregano, toss, introduce in your Air Fryer and cook at 380 ° F for 15 minutes.
2. Divide between plates and serve as a side dish.

Gold Potatoes and Bell Pepper Mix

Preparation Time: 10 minutes

Cooking Time: 25 minutes

Servings:

Ingredients

- 4 gold potatoes, cubed
- 1 yellow onion, chopped
- 2 teaspoons olive oil
- 1 green bell pepper, chopped
- Salt and black pepper to the taste
- ½ teaspoon thyme, dried

Directions:

1. Heat up your Air Fryer at 350 ° F, add oil, heat it up, add onion, bell pepper, salt and pepper, stir and cook for 5 minutes.

2. Add potatoes and thyme, stir, cover and cook at 360 °F for 20 minutes.
3. Divide between plates and serve as a side dish.

Eggplant Salad

Preparation time: 10 minutes

Cooking time: 50 minutes

Servings: 3

Ingredients:

- 2 lbs. firm young eggplant
- 2½ Tbs. brown sugar
- 2 Tbs. onion, minced
- 2 cloves garlic, minced
- 1 Tbs. olive oil
- 2 Tbs. cider vinegar
- 2 generous tsp. grated fresh ginger
- 2 tsp. fresh lemon juice

Directions:

1. Prick the eggplants in several places with a fork and roast them in a 400 degree oven until they are quite soft.
2. When the eggplants are cool enough to handle, cut them in half and scrape the pulp carefully out of the skin.

3. If the seeds are dark brown and starting to separate from the eggplant, plant, they will be bitter and must be removed (meaning it wasn't quite young or fresh enough).
4. If the seeds are pale and small, leave them. Drain the eggplant pulp thoroughly in a large sieve and mince it.
5. Combine the minced eggplant in a bowl with all the remaining ingredients, mix well, and chill several hours.
6. Serve small portions of the chilled eggplant on lettuce leaves as a first course, or with unsalted crackers as a dip.

Savory Spanish Rice

Servings: 10

Preparation time: 3 hours and 10 minutes

Ingredients:

- 1 cup of long grain rice, uncooked
- 1/2 cup of chopped green bell pepper
- 14 ounce of diced tomatoes
- 1/2 cup of chopped white onion
- 1 teaspoon of minced garlic
- 1/2 teaspoon of salt
- 1 teaspoon of red chili powder
- 1 teaspoon of ground cumin
- 4-ounce of tomato puree
- 8 fluid ounce of water

Directions:

1. Grease a 6-quarts slow cooker with a non-stick cooking spray and add all the ingredients into it.
2. Stir properly and cover the top.

3. Plug in the slow cooker; adjust the cooking time to 5 hours and let it cook on the high heat setting or until the rice absorbs all the liquid.
4. Serve right away.

Tastiest Barbecued Tofu and Vegetables

Servings: 4

Preparation time: 4 hours 15 minutes

Ingredients:

- 14-ounce of extra-firm tofu, pressed and drained
- 2 medium-sized zucchini, steamed and diced
- 1/2 large green bell pepper, cored and cubed
- 3 stalks of broccoli stalks
- 8 ounce of sliced water chestnuts
- 1 small white onion, peeled and minced
- 1 1/2 teaspoon of minced garlic
- 2 teaspoons of minced ginger
- 1 1/2 teaspoon of salt
- 1/8 teaspoon of ground black pepper
- 1/4 teaspoon of crushed red pepper
- 1/4 teaspoon of five spice powder
- 2 teaspoons of molasses
- 1 tablespoon of whole-grain mustard
- 1/4 teaspoon of vegan Worcestershire sauce

- 8 ounces of tomato sauce
- 1/4 cup of hoisin sauce
- 1 tablespoon of soy sauce
- 2 tablespoons of apple cider vinegar
- 2 tablespoons of water

Directions:

1. Take a 6-quarts slow cooker, grease it with a non-stick cooking spray and set it aside until it is required.
2. Place a medium-sized non-stick skillet pan over an average heat, add the oil and let it heat.
3. Cut the tofu into 1/2 inch pieces and add it to the skillet pan in a single layer.
4. Cook for 3 minutes per sides and then transfer it to the prepared slow cooker.
5. When the tofu turns brown, place it into the pan, add the onion, garlic, ginger and cook for 3 to 5 minutes or until the onions are softened.
6. Add the remaining ingredients into the pan except for the vegetables which are the broccoli stalks, zucchini, bell pepper and water chestnuts.
7. Stir until it mixes properly and cook for 2 minutes or until the mixture starts bubbling.
8. Transfer this mixture into the slow cooker and stir properly.

9. Cover the top, plug in the slow cooker; adjust the cooking time to 3 hours and let it cook on the high heat setting or until it is cooked thoroughly.
10. In the meantime, trim the broccoli stalks and cut it into 1/4 inch pieces.
11. When the tofu is cooked thoroughly, put it into the slow cooker; add the broccoli stalks and the remaining vegetables.
12. Stir until it mixes properly and then return the top to cover it.
13. Continue cooking for 1 hour at the high heat setting or until the vegetables are tender.
14. Serve right away with rice.

Super tasty Vegetarian Chili

Servings: 6

Preparation time: 2 hours and 10 minutes

Ingredients:

- 16-ounce of vegetarian baked beans
- 16 ounce of cooked chickpeas
- 16 ounce of cooked kidney beans
- 15 ounce of cooked corn
- 1 medium-sized green bell pepper, cored and chopped
- 2 stalks of celery, peeled and chopped
- 12 ounce of chopped tomatoes
- 1 medium-sized white onion, peeled and chopped
- 1 teaspoon of minced garlic
- 1 teaspoon of salt
- 1 tablespoon of red chili powder
- 1 tablespoon of dried oregano
- 1 tablespoon of dried basil
- 1 tablespoon of dried parsley
- 18-ounce of black bean soup
- 4-ounce of tomato puree

Directions:

1. Take a 6-quarts slow cooker, grease it with a non-stick cooking spray and place all the ingredients into it.
2. Stir properly and cover the top.
3. Plug in the slow cooker; adjust the cooking time to 2 hours and let it cook on the high heat setting or until it is cooked thoroughly.
4. Serve right away.

Comforting Chickpea Tagine

Servings: 6

Preparation time: 4 hours and 15 minutes

Ingredients:

- 14 ounce of cooked chickpeas
- 12 dried apricots
- 1 red bell pepper, cored and sliced
- 1 small butternut squash, peeled, cored and chopped
- 2 zucchini, stemmed and chopped
- 1 medium-sized white onion, peeled and chopped
- 1 teaspoon of minced garlic
- 1 teaspoon of ground ginger
- 1 1/2 teaspoon of salt
- 1 teaspoon of ground black pepper
- 1 teaspoon of ground cumin
- 2 teaspoon of paprika
- 1 teaspoon of harissa paste
- 2 teaspoon of honey
- 2 tablespoons of olive oil
- 1 pound of passata
- 1/4 cup of chopped coriander

Directions:

1. Take a 6-quarts slow cooker, grease it with a non-stick cooking spray and place the chickpeas, apricots, bell pepper, butternut squash, zucchini and onion into it.
2. Sprinkle it with salt, black pepper and set it aside until it is called for.
3. Place a large non-stick skillet pan over an average temperature of heat; add the oil, garlic, cumin and paprika.
4. Stir properly and cook for 1 minutes or until it starts producing fragrance.
5. Then pour in the harissa paste, honey, passata and boil the mixture.
6. When the mixture is done boiling, pour this mixture over the vegetables in the slow cooker and cover it with the lid.
7. Plug in the slow cooker; adjust the cooking time to 4 hours and let it cook on the high heat setting or until the vegetables gets tender.
8. When done, add the seasoning, garnish it with the coriander and serve right away.

Falafel

Preparation time: 10 minutes

Cooking time: 30 minutes

Servings: 4

Ingredients:

- ¼ cup and 1 tablespoon olive oil
- 1 cup chickpeas, cooked
- ½ cup chopped parsley
- ½ cup chopped red onion
- ½ cup chopped cilantro
- 2 teaspoons minced garlic
- ½ teaspoon ground black pepper
- ¼ teaspoon ground cinnamon
- 1 teaspoon of sea salt
- ½ teaspoon ground cumin

Directions:

1. Place all the ingredients in a food processor, reserving ¼ cup oil, and pulse until smooth.

2. Shape the mixture into small patties, place them on a rimmed baking sheet, greased with remaining oil and bake for 30 minutes until cooked and roasted on both sides, turning halfway through.
3. Serve straight away.

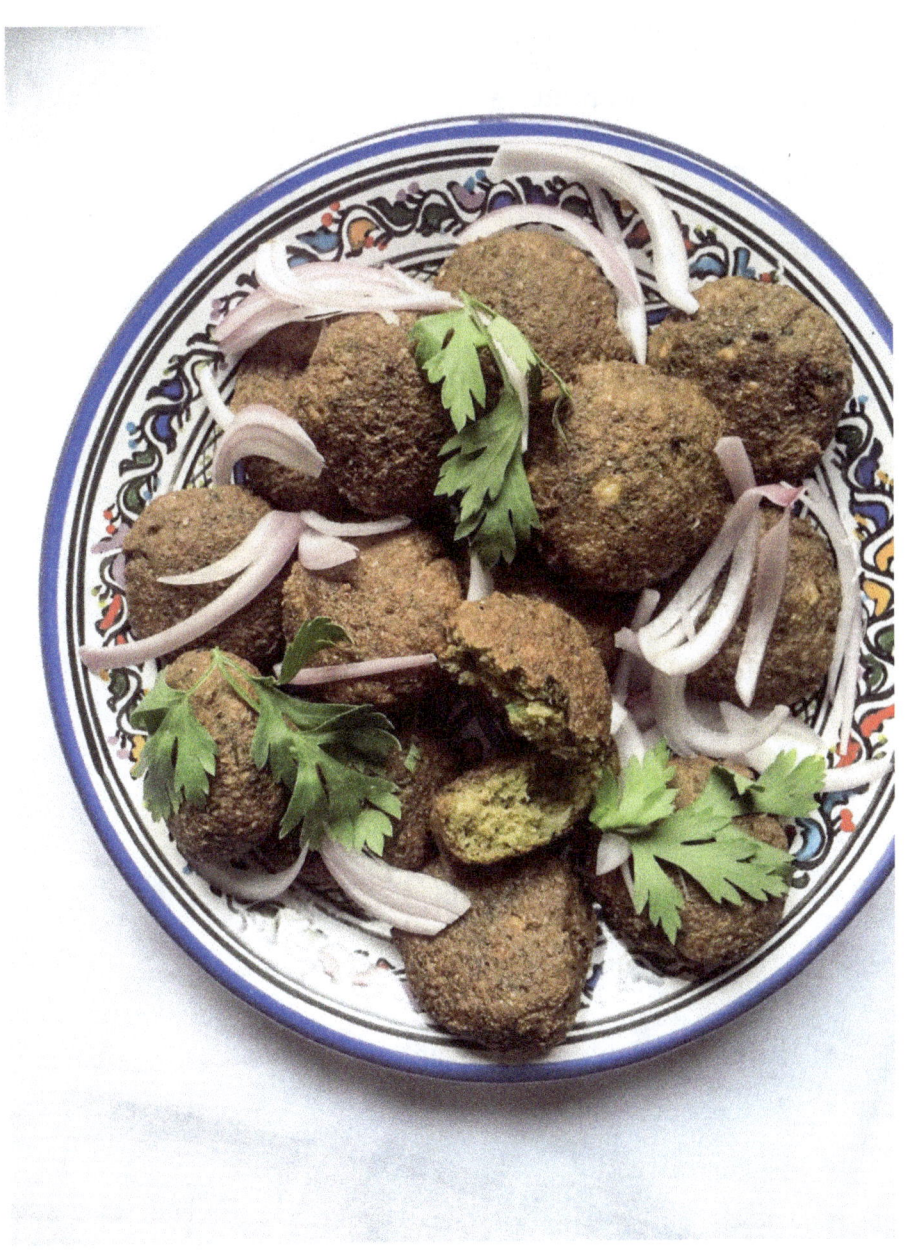

Lebanese Bean Salad

Preparation time: 10 minutes

Cooking time: 0 minute

Servings: 4

Ingredients:

For the Salad:

- 1 ½ cups cooked chickpeas
- 3 cups cooked kidney beans
- 1 small red onion, peeled, diced
- 1 medium cucumber, peeled, deseeded, diced
- 2 stalks celery, chopped
- ¾ cup chopped parsley
- 2 tablespoons chopped dill

For the Dressing:

- 1 ½ teaspoon minced garlic
- ¾ teaspoon salt
- ¼ cup olive oil
- 1/8 teaspoon red pepper flakes
- ¼ cup lemon juice

Directions:

1. Prepare the dressing and for this, place all of its ingredients in a bowl and whisk until combined.
2. Take a large bowl, place all the ingredients for the salad in it, drizzle with the dressing and toss until combined.
3. Serve straight away.

Lentil Soup

Preparation time: 10 minutes

Cooking time: 50 minutes

Servings: 4

Ingredients:

- 1 cup green lentils
- 1 medium white onion, peeled, chopped
- 1 cup chopped kale leaves
- 28 ounces diced tomatoes
- 2 carrots, peeled, chopped
- 2 teaspoons minced garlic
- 1 teaspoon curry powder
- ¼ teaspoon ground black pepper
- 1 teaspoon salt
- 2 teaspoons ground cumin
- 1/8 teaspoon red pepper flakes
- ½ teaspoon dried thyme
- ¼ cup olive oil
- 4 cups vegetable broth
- 1 tablespoon lemon juice

- 2 cups of water

Directions:

1. Take a large pot, place it over medium heat, add 1 tablespoon oil and when hot, add onion and carrot and cook for 5 minutes until softened.
2. Then stir in garlic, curry powder, cumin and thyme, cook for 1 minute, then stir in tomatoes and cook for 3 minutes.
3. Add lentils, pour in water and broth, season with black pepper, salt, and red pepper and bring the mixture to a boil.
4. Switch heat to medium-low, simmer lentils for 30 minutes, then puree half of the soup, return it into the pan, stir in kale and cook for 5 minutes until softened.
5. Drizzle with lemon juice and serve straight away.

Quinoa and Black Beans

Preparation time: 10 minutes

Cooking time: 35 minutes

Servings: 4

Ingredients:

- 3/4 cup quinoa
- 30 ounces cooked black beans
- 1 medium white onion, peeled, chopped
- 1 ½ teaspoon minced garlic
- 1 cup frozen corn kernels
- ¼ teaspoon ground black pepper
- 1/3 teaspoon salt
- 1 teaspoon ground cumin
- 1/4 teaspoon cayenne
- 1 teaspoon olive oil
- 1 1/2 cups vegetable broth
- 1/2 cup chopped cilantro

Directions:

1. Take a saucepan, place it over medium heat, add oil and when hot, add onion and garlic, and cook for 10 minutes until softened.
2. Add quinoa, pour in the broth, stir in all the seasoning, then bring the mixture to a boil, switch heat to medium-low level and simmer for 20 minutes until the quinoa has absorbed all the liquid.
3. Add corn, stir until mixed, cook for 5 minutes until heated, and then stir in beans until mixed.
4. Garnish with cilantro and serve.

Stuffed Peppers

Preparation time: 10 minutes

Cooking time: 20 minutes

Servings: 4

Ingredients:

- 2 green onions, sliced
- 2 green bell peppers, halved, cored
- 1 large tomato, diced
- 1/2 cup Arborio rice, cooked
- ¼ teaspoon ground black pepper
- 1 teaspoon Italian seasoning
- 1 teaspoon salt
- 1 teaspoon dried basil
- 1 tablespoon olive oil
- 1 cup of water
- 1/2 cup crumbled vegan feta cheese

Directions:

1. Prepare the peppers and for this, cut them in half, then remove the seeds and roast them on a greased baking sheet for 20 minutes at 400 degrees F until tender.
2. Meanwhile, heat oil in a skillet pan over medium-high heat and when hot, add onion, season with seasonings and herbs, and cook for 3 minutes.
3. Add tomatoes, stir well, cook for 5 minutes, then stir in rice and cook for 3 minutes until heated.
4. When done, remove the pan from heat, stir in cheese, and stuff the mixture into roasted peppers.
5. Serve straight away.

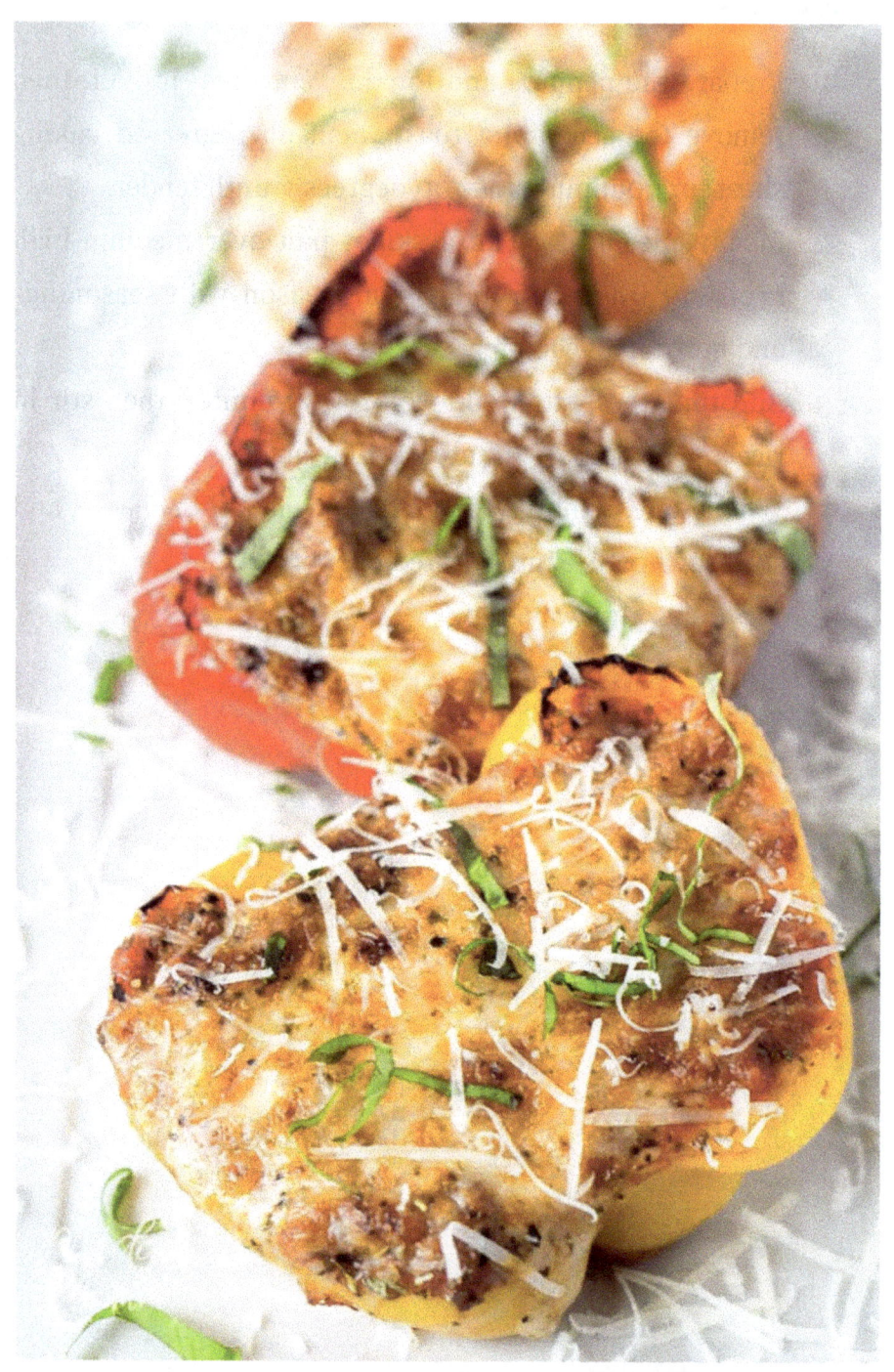

Vegetable Barley Soup

Preparation time: 5 minutes

Cooking time: 15 minutes

Servings: 8

Ingredients:

- 1 cup barley
- 14.5 ounces diced tomatoes with juice
- 2 large carrots, chopped
- 15 ounces cooked chickpeas
- 2 stalks celery, chopped
- 1 zucchini, chopped
- 1 medium white onion, peeled, chopped
- 1/2 teaspoon ground black pepper
- 1 teaspoon garlic powder
- 1 teaspoon curry powder
- 1 teaspoon salt
- 1 teaspoon paprika
- 1 teaspoon white sugar
- 1 teaspoon dried parsley
- 1 teaspoon Worcestershire sauce

- 3 bay leaves
- 2 quarts vegetable broth

Directions:

1. Place all the ingredients in a pot, stir until mixed, place it over medium-high heat and bring the mixture to a boil.
2. Switch heat to medium level, simmer the soup for 90 minutes until cooked, and when done, remove bay leaf from it.
3. Serve straight away.

Asparagus Rice Pilaf

Preparation time: 10 minutes

Cooking time: 35 minutes

Servings: 4

Ingredients:

- 1 1/4 cups rice
- 1/2 pound asparagus, diced, boiled
- 2 ounces spaghetti, whole-grain, broken
- 1/4 cup minced white onion
- 1/2 teaspoon minced garlic
- 1/2 cup cashew halves
- ¼ teaspoon ground black pepper
- ½ teaspoon salt
- 1/4 cup vegan butter
- 2 1/4 cups vegetable broth

Directions:

1. Take a saucepan, place it over medium-low heat, add butter and when it melts, stir in spaghetti and cook for 3 minutes until golden brown.

2. Add onion and garlic, cook for 2 minutes until tender, then stir in rice, cook for 5 minutes, pour in the broth, season with salt and black pepper and bring it to a boil.
3. Switch heat to medium level, cook for 20 minutes, then add cashews and asparagus and stir until combined.
4. Serve straight away.

Quinoa and Black Bean Chili

Preparation time: 10 minutes

Cooking time: 32 minutes

Servings: 10

Ingredients:

- 1 cup quinoa, cooked
- 38 ounces cooked black beans
- 1 medium white onion, peeled, chopped
- 1 cup of frozen corn
- 1 green bell pepper, deseeded, chopped
- 1 zucchini, chopped
- 1 tablespoon minced chipotle peppers in adobo sauce
- 1 red bell pepper, deseeded, chopped
- 1 jalapeno pepper, deseeded, minced
- 28 ounces crushed tomatoes
- 2 teaspoons minced garlic
- 1/3 teaspoon ground black pepper
- ¾ teaspoon salt
- 1 teaspoon dried oregano
- 1 tablespoon red chili powder

- 1 tablespoon ground cumin
- 1 tablespoon olive oil
- 1/4 cup chopped cilantro

Directions:

1. Take a large pot, place it over medium heat, add oil and when hot, add onion and cook for 5 minutes.
2. Then stir in garlic, cumin, and chili powder, cook for 1 minute, add remaining ingredients except for corn and quinoa, stir well and simmer for 20 minutes at medium-low heat until cooked.
3. Then stir in corn and quinoa, cook for 5 minutes until hot and then top with cilantro.
4. Serve straight away.

Quinoa with Chickpeas and Tomatoes

Preparation time: 10 minutes

Cooking time: 0 minute

Servings: 6

Ingredients:

- 1 tomato, chopped
- 1 cup quinoa, cooked
- ½ teaspoon minced garlic
- ¼ teaspoon ground black pepper
- ½ teaspoon salt
- 1/2 teaspoon ground cumin
- 4 teaspoons olive oil
- 3 tablespoons lime juice
- 1/2 teaspoon chopped parsley

Directions:

1. Take a large bowl, place all the ingredients in it, except for the parsley, and stir until mixed.
2. Garnish with parsley and serve straight away.

Zucchini Risotto

Preparation time: 10 minutes

Cooking time: 30 minutes

Servings: 6

Ingredients:

- 2 cups Arborio rice
- 10 sun-dried tomatoes, chopped
- 1 medium white onion, peeled, chopped
- 1 tablespoon chopped basil leaves
- 1/2 medium zucchini, sliced
- 1 teaspoon dried thyme
- 1/3 teaspoon ground black pepper
- 1 tablespoon vegan butter
- 6 tablespoons grated vegan Parmesan cheese
- 7 cups vegetable broth, hot

Directions:

1. Take a large pot, place it over medium heat, add butter and when it melts, add onion and cook for 2 minutes.

2. Stir in rice, cook for another 2 minutes until toasted, and then stir in broth, 1 cup at a time until absorbed completely and creamy mixture comes together.
3. Then stir in remaining ingredients until combined, taste to adjust seasoning and serve

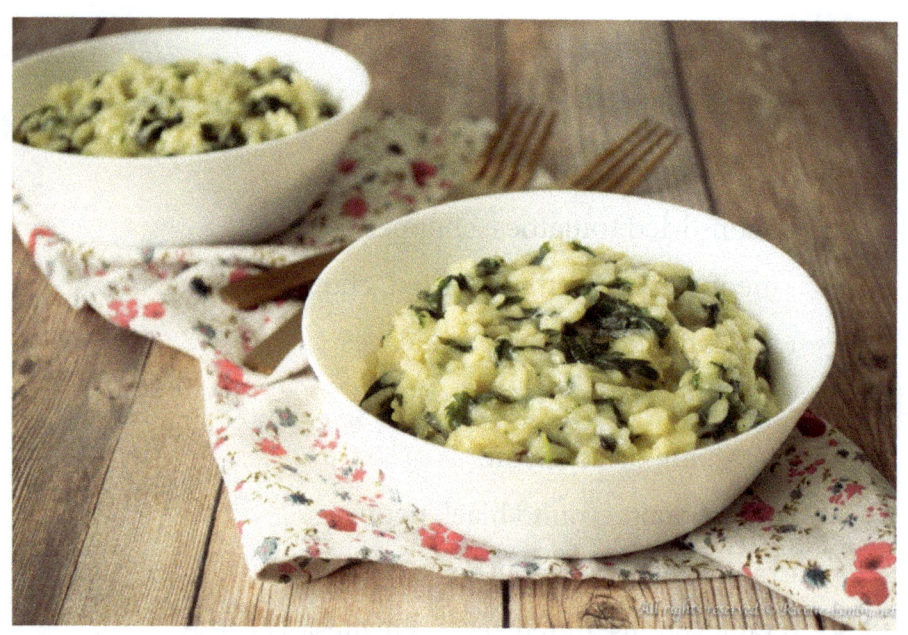

Tomato Barley Soup

Preparation time: 10 minutes

Cooking time: 40 minutes

Servings: 6

Ingredients:

- 1/4 cup barley
- 1 cup chopped celery
- 14.5 ounces peeled and diced tomatoes
- 1 cup chopped white onions
- 2 tomatoes, diced
- 1 cup chopped carrots
- 2 teaspoons minced garlic
- 1/8 teaspoon ground black pepper
- 1 teaspoon salt
- 2 tablespoons olive oil
- 2 1/2 cups water
- 10.75 ounces chicken broth

Directions:

1. Take a large saucepan, place it over medium heat, add onion, carrot, and celery, stir in garlic and cook for 10 minutes until tender.
2. Then add remaining ingredients, stir until combined, and bring the mixture to a boil.
3. Switch heat to the level, simmer the soup for 40 minutes and then serve straight away.

Lemony Quinoa

Preparation time: 10 minutes

Cooking time: 0 minute

Servings: 6

Ingredients:

- 1 cup quinoa, cooked
- 1/4 of medium red onion, peeled, chopped
- 1 bunch of parsley, chopped
- 2 stalks of celery, chopped
- 1/4 teaspoon of sea salt
- 1/4 teaspoon cayenne pepper
- 1/2 teaspoon ground cumin
- 1/4 cup lemon juice
- 1/4 cup pine nuts, toasted

Directions:

1. Take a large bowl, place all the ingredients in it, and stir until combined.
2. Serve straight away.

Brown Rice, Broccoli, and Walnut

Preparation time: 5 minutes

Cooking time: 18 minutes

Servings: 4

Ingredients:

- 1 cup of brown rice
- 1 medium white onion, peeled, chopped
- 1 pound broccoli florets
- ½ cup chopped walnuts, toasted
- ½ teaspoon minced garlic
- ⅛ teaspoon ground black pepper
- ½ teaspoon salt
- 1 tablespoon vegan butter
- 1 cup vegetable broth
- 1 cup shredded vegan cheddar cheese

Directions:

1. Take a saucepan, place it over medium heat, add butter and when it melts, add onion and garlic and cook for 3 minutes.
2. Stir in rice, pour in the broth, bring the mixture to boil, then switch heat to medium-low level and simmer until rice has absorbed all the liquid.
3. Meanwhile, take a casserole dish, place broccoli florets in it, sprinkle with salt and black pepper, cover with a plastic wrap and microwave for 5 minutes until tender.
4. Place cooked rice in a dish, top with broccoli, sprinkle with nuts and cheese, and then serve.

Broccoli and Rice Stir Fry

Preparation time: 5 minutes

Cooking time: 10 minutes

Servings: 8

Ingredients:

- 16 ounces frozen broccoli florets, thawed
- 3 green onions, diced
- ½ teaspoon salt
- ¼ teaspoon ground black pepper
- 2 tablespoons soy sauce
- 1 tablespoon olive oil
- 1 ½ cups white rice, cooked

Directions:

1. Take a skillet pan, place it over medium heat, add broccoli, and cook for 5 minutes until tender-crisp.
2. Then add scallion and other ingredients, toss until well mixed and cook for 2 minutes until hot.
3. Serve straight away.

Coconut Rice

Preparation time: 10 minutes

Cooking time: 25 minutes

Servings: 7

Ingredients:

- 2 1/2 cups white rice
- 1/8 teaspoon salt
- 40 ounces coconut milk, unsweetened

Directions:

1. Take a large saucepan, place it over medium heat, add all the ingredients in it and stir until mixed.
2. Bring the mixture to a boil, then switch heat to medium-low level and simmer rice for 25 minutes until tender and all the liquid is absorbed.
3. Serve straight away.

Brown Rice Pilaf

Preparation time: 5 minutes

Cooking time: 25 minutes

Servings: 4

Ingredients:

- 1 cup cooked chickpeas
- 3/4 cup brown rice, cooked
- 1/4 cup chopped cashews
- 2 cups sliced mushrooms
- 2 carrots, sliced
- ½ teaspoon minced garlic
- 1 1/2 cups chopped white onion
- 3 tablespoons vegan butter
- ½ teaspoon salt
- ¼ teaspoon ground black pepper
- 1/4 cup chopped parsley

Directions:

1. Take a large skillet pan, place it over medium heat, add butter and when it melts, add onions and cook them for 5 minutes until softened.
2. Then add carrots and garlic, cook for 5 minutes, add mushrooms, cook for 10 minutes until browned, add chickpeas and cook for another minute.
3. When done, remove the pan from heat, add nuts, parsley, salt and black pepper, toss until mixed, and garnish with parsley.
4. Serve straight away.

Vegan Curried Rice

Preparation time: 5 minutes

Cooking time: 25 minutes

Servings: 4

Ingredients:

- 1 cup white rice
- 1 tablespoon minced garlic
- 1 tablespoon ground curry powder
- 1/3 teaspoon ground black pepper
- 1 tablespoon red chili powder
- 1 tablespoon ground cumin
- 2 tablespoons olive oil
- 1 tablespoon soy sauce
- 1 cup vegetable broth

Directions:

1. Take a saucepan, place it over low heat, add oil and when hot, add garlic and cook for 3 minutes.
2. Then stir in all spices, cook for 1 minute until fragrant, pour in the broth, and switch heat to a high level.

3. Stir in soy sauce, bring the mixture to boil, add rice, stir until mixed, then switch heat to the low level and simmer for 20 minutes until rice is tender and all the liquid has absorbed.
4. Serve straight away.

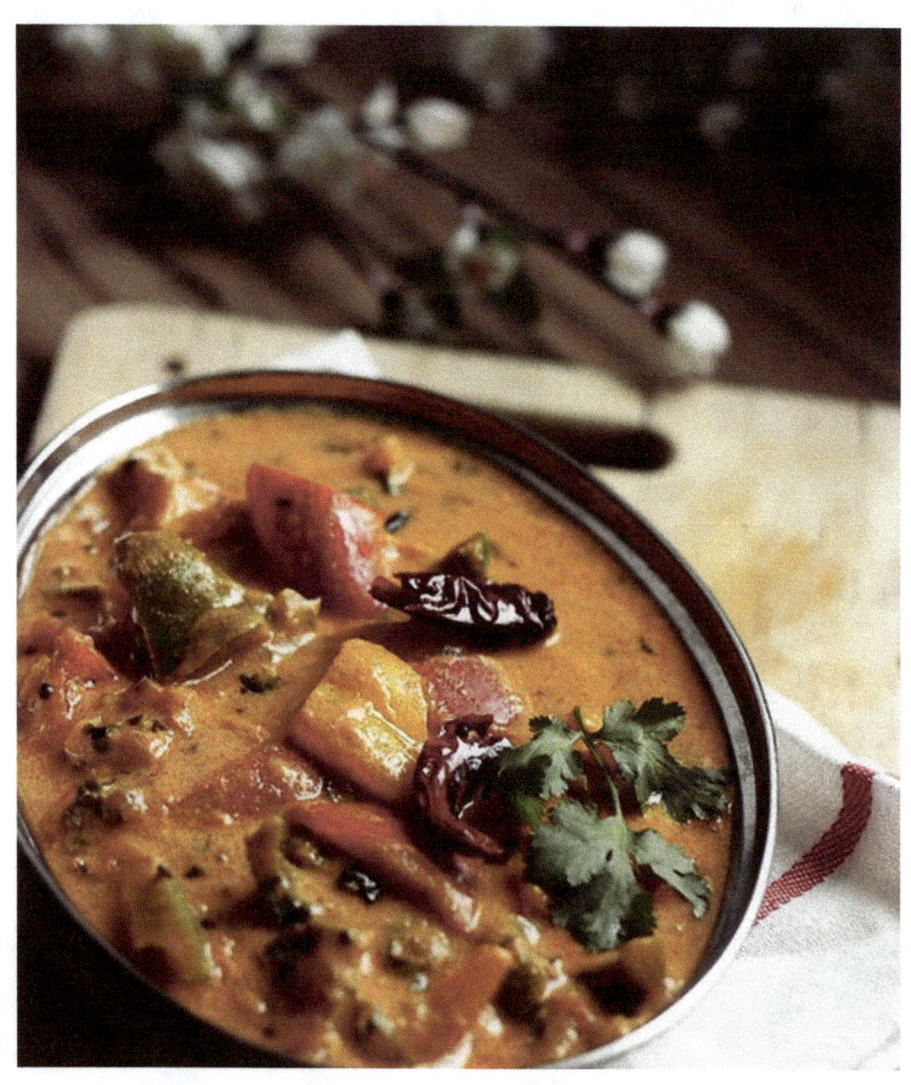

Coconut Curry Lentils

Preparation time: 10 minutes

Cooking time: 40 minutes

Servings: 4

Ingredients:

- 1 cup brown lentils
- 1 small white onion, peeled, chopped
- 1 teaspoon minced garlic
- 1 teaspoon grated ginger
- 3 cups baby spinach
- 1 tablespoon curry powder
- 2 tablespoons olive oil
- 13 ounces coconut milk, unsweetened
- 2 cups vegetable broth

For Serving:

- 4 cups cooked rice
- 1/4 cup chopped cilantro

Directions:

1. Place a large pot over medium heat, add oil and when hot, add ginger and garlic and cook for 1 minute until fragrant.
2. Add onion, cook for 5 minutes, stir in curry powder, cook for 1 minute until toasted, add lentils and pour in broth.
3. Switch heat to medium-high level, bring the mixture to a boil, then switch heat to the low level and simmer for 20 minutes until tender and all the liquid is absorbed.
4. Pour in milk, stir until combined, turn heat to medium level, and simmer for 10 minutes until thickened.
5. Then remove the pot from heat, stir in spinach, let it stand for 5 minutes until its leaves wilts and then top with cilantro.
6. Serve lentils with rice.

Chard Wraps With Millet

Preparation time: 25 minutes

Cooking time: 0 minute

Servings: 4

Ingredients:

- 1 carrot, cut into ribbons
- 1/2 cup millet, cooked
- 1/2 of a large cucumber, cut into ribbons
- 1/2 cup chickpeas, cooked
- 1 cup sliced cabbage
- 1/3 cup hummus
- Mint leaves as needed for topping
- Hemp seeds as needed for topping
- 1 bunch of Swiss rainbow chard

Directions:

1. Spread hummus on one side of chard, place some of millet, vegetables, and chickpeas on it, sprinkle with some mint leaves and hemp seeds and wrap it like a burrito.
2. Serve straight away.

Rice Stuffed Jalapeños

Preparation time: 5 minutes

Cooking time: 15 minutes

Servings: 6

Ingredients:

- 3 medium-sized potatoes, peeled, cubed, boiled
- 2 large carrots, peeled, chopped, boiled
- 3 tablespoons water
- 1/4 teaspoon onion powder
- 1 teaspoons salt
- 1/2 cup nutritional yeast
- 1/4 teaspoon garlic powder
- 1 lime, juiced
- 3 tablespoons water
- Cooked rice as needed
- 3 jalapeños pepper, halved
- 1 red bell pepper, sliced, for garnish
- ½ cup vegetable broth

Directions:

1. Place boiled vegetables in a food processor, pour in broth and pulse until smooth.
2. Add garlic powder, onion powder, salt, water, and lime juice, pulse until combined, then add yeast and blend until smooth.
3. Tip the mixture in a bowl, add rice, and stir until incorporated.
4. Cut each jalapeno into half lengthwise, brush them with oil, season them with some salt, stuff them with rice mixture and bake them for 20 minutes at 400 degrees F until done.
5. Serve straight away.

Lentil and Wild Rice Soup

Preparation time: 10 minutes

Cooking time: 40 minutes

Servings: 4

Ingredients:

- 1/2 cup cooked mixed beans
- 12 ounces cooked lentils
- 2 stalks of celery, sliced
- 1 1/2 cup mixed wild rice, cooked
- 1 large sweet potato, peeled, chopped
- 1/2 medium butternut, peeled, chopped
- 4 medium carrots, peeled, sliced
- 1 medium onion, peeled, diced
- 10 cherry tomatoes
- 1/2 red chili, deseeded, diced
- 1 ½ teaspoon minced garlic
- 1/2 teaspoon salt
- 2 teaspoons mixed dried herbs
- 1 teaspoon coconut oil
- 2 cups vegetable broth

Directions:

1. Take a large pot, place it over medium-high heat, add oil and when it melts, add onion and cook for 5 minutes.
2. Stir in garlic and chili, cook for 3 minutes, then add remaining vegetables, pour in the broth, stir and bring the mixture to a boil.
3. Switch heat to medium-low heat, cook the soup for 20 minutes, then stir in remaining ingredients and continue cooking for 10 minutes until soup has reached to desired thickness.
4. Serve straight away.

Black Beans and Cauliflower Rice

Preparation time: 10 minutes

Cooking time: 20 minutes

Servings: 4

Ingredients:

- 3 cups cauliflower rice
- 15.5 ounces cooked black beans
- 1/2 cup diced red bell pepper
- 1/2 cup chopped onion
- 3 tablespoons chopped pickled jalapeno
- 1 ½ teaspoon minced garlic
- ¼ teaspoon ground black pepper
- 1/3 teaspoon sea salt
- 1/4 teaspoon ground cayenne pepper
- 2 tablespoons olive oil
- 1/2 cup diced parsley

Directions:

1. Take a large skillet pan, place it over medium heat, add oil and garlic and cook for 2 minutes.
2. Then add onion and bell pepper, season with black pepper, salt, and cayenne pepper, cook for 5 minutes, then stir in jalapeno pepper and top with cauliflower rice.
3. Season with salt and black pepper, cook for 7 minutes, turning halfway, then add beans and cook for 2 minutes until hot.
4. Garnish with parsley and serve.

Black Bean and Quinoa Salad

Preparation time: 10 minutes

Cooking time: 0 minute

Servings: 10

Ingredients:

- 15 ounces cooked black beans
- 1 medium red bell pepper, cored, chopped
- 1 cup quinoa, cooked
- 1 medium green bell pepper, cored, chopped
- 1/2 cup vegan feta cheese, crumbled

Directions:

1. Place all the ingredients in a large bowl, except for cheese, and stir until incorporated.
2. Top the salad with cheese and serve straight away.

Coconut Chickpea Curry

Preparation time: 10 minutes

Cooking time: 30 minutes

Servings: 4

Ingredients:

- 2 teaspoons coconut flour
- 16 ounces cooked chickpeas
- 14 ounces tomatoes, diced
- 1 large red onion, sliced
- 1 ½ teaspoon minced garlic
- ½ teaspoon of sea salt
- 1 teaspoon curry powder
- 1/3 teaspoon ground black pepper
- 1 ½ tablespoons garam masala
- 1/4 teaspoon cumin
- 1 small lime, juiced
- 13.5 ounces coconut milk, unsweetened
- 2 tablespoons coconut oil

Directions:

1. Take a large pot, place it over medium-high heat, add oil and when it melts, add onions and tomatoes, season with salt and black pepper and cook for 5 minutes.
2. Switch heat to medium-low level, cook for 10 minutes until tomatoes have released their liquid, then add chickpeas and stir in garlic, curry powder, garam masala, and cumin until combined.
3. Stir in milk and flour, bring the mixture to boil, then switch heat to medium heat and simmer the curry for 12 minutes until cooked.
4. Taste to adjust seasoning, drizzle with lime juice, and serve

Zoodles with White Beans

Preparation time: 10 minutes

Cooking time: 20 minutes

Servings: 4

Ingredients:

- 15 ounces cooked cannellini beans
- 2 medium zucchini, spiralized into noodles
- 3 teaspoons minced garlic
- 1 cup chopped Roma tomatoes
- 2/3 teaspoon salt
- 1/8 teaspoon red pepper flakes
- 1/4 cup olive oil
- 1/4 cup chopped parsley
- 4 ounces whole-grain spaghetti, cooked

Directions:

1. Cook the pasta, drain it, transfer it into a bowl, add zucchini noodles and toss until mixed.

2. Take a pot, place it over low heat, add oil, garlic, and red pepper flakes, stir until cook for 5 minutes until garlic is golden brown.
3. Then add all the ingredients, except for parsley and salt, toss until mixed and cook for 5 minutes until thoroughly heated.
4. When done, season with salt, top with parsley and serve.

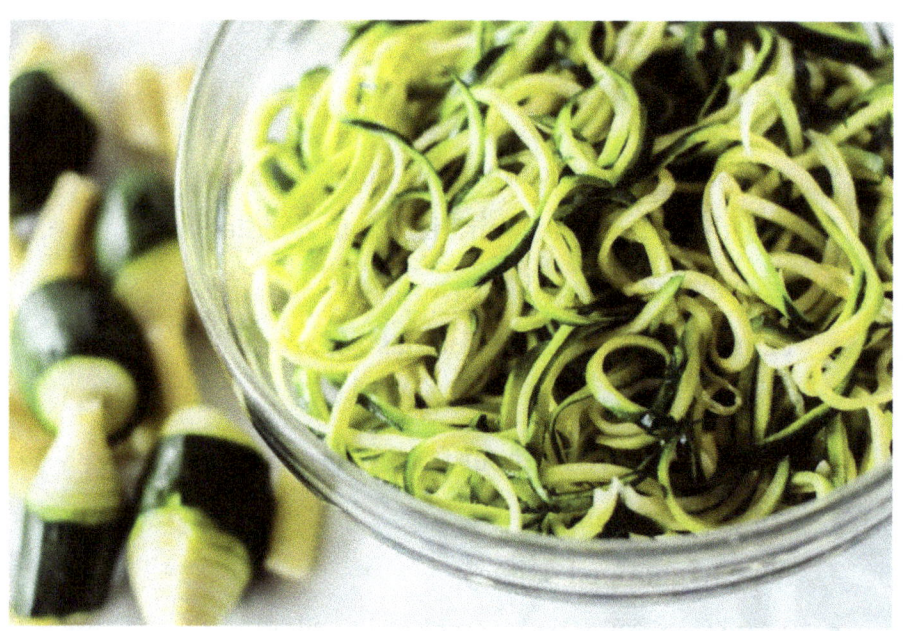

Pasta with Kidney Bean Sauce

Preparation time: 5 minutes

Cooking time: 15 minutes

Servings: 4

Ingredients:

- 12 ounces cooked kidney beans
- 7 ounces whole-wheat pasta, cooked
- 1 medium white onion, peeled, diced
- 1 cup arugula
- 2 tablespoons tomato paste
- 1 teaspoon minced garlic
- ½ teaspoon smoked paprika
- 1 teaspoon dried oregano
- ½ teaspoon cayenne pepper
- 1/3 teaspoon ground black pepper
- 2/3 teaspoon salt
- 2 tablespoons balsamic vinegar

Directions:

1. Take a large skillet pan, place it over medium-high heat, add onion and garlic, splash with some water and cook for 5 minutes.
2. Then add remaining ingredients, except for pasta and arugula, stir until mixed and cook for 10 minutes until thickened.
3. When done, mash with the fork, top with arugula and serve with pasta.
4. Serve straight away

Chickpea Shakshuka

Preparation time: 5 minutes

Cooking time: 30 minutes

Servings: 6

Ingredients:

- 22 ounces cooked chickpeas
- 1/2 cup diced white onion
- 5 green olives
- 1/2 medium red bell pepper, chopped
- 1 1/2 Tbsp minced garlic
- 1 Tbsp coconut sugar
- 2 teaspoons red chili powder
- 2 teaspoons smoked paprika
- 1/8 teaspoon cayenne pepper
- 1 teaspoon salt
- 3 Tbsp tomato paste
- 1 tsp ground cumin
- 1/4 teaspoon ground cinnamon
- 1/8 teaspoon cardamom
- 1/8 teaspoon coriander

- 28-ounces tomato puree
- 1 Tbsp avocado oil

Directions:

1. Take a large skillet pan, place it over medium heat, add oil and when hot, add garlic, onion and bell pepper and cook for 5 minutes until fragrant.
2. Then stir in the tomato puree and tomato paste, stir in all the spices until combined, bring the mixture to simmer, and cook for 3 minutes.
3. Add olives and chickpeas, stir to combine, switch heat to medium-low level and simmer for 20 minutes until cooked.
4. Serve straight away.

Avocado Burrito Bowl

Preparation time: 5 minutes

Cooking time: 10 minutes

Servings: 4

Ingredients:

- 1 cup brown rice, cooked

For Marinated Kale:

- 1 bunch of kale, chopped
- ¼ cup lime juice
- 2 tablespoons olive oil
- ½ jalapeño, deseeded, chopped
- ½ teaspoon cumin
- ¼ teaspoon salt

For Avocado Salsa:

- 1 avocado, pitted, sliced
- ½ cup cilantro leaves
- ½ cup salsa verde
- 2 tablespoons lime juice

For Seasoned Black Beans:

- 1/3 cup chopped red onion
- 4 cups cooked black beans
- 1 ½ teaspoon minced garlic
- ¼ teaspoon cayenne pepper
- ¼ teaspoon red chili powder
- 1 tablespoon olive oil

For Garnish:

- 6 Cherry tomatoes, sliced into thin rounds
- 4 teaspoons hot sauce

Directions:

1. Prepare kale and for this, place all its ingredients in a large bowl and toss until combined, set aside until required.
2. Prepare the salsa, and for this, place all its ingredients in a blender, process until smooth, and set aside until required.
3. Prepare beans and for this, take a saucepan, place it over medium-low heat, add oil and when hot, add onion and garlic and cook for 2 minutes.
4. Then add remaining ingredients, stir until mixed and cook for 7 minutes until beans are heated and tender.

5. Top rice with beans, kale, and salsa, drizzle with hot sauce and serve with tomatoes.

Sweet Potato and Bean Burgers

Preparation time: 10 minutes

Cooking time: 50 minutes

Servings: 8

Ingredients:

- 1 cup oats, old-fashioned, ground
- 1 ½ pounds sweet potatoes
- 1 cup cooked millet
- 15 ounces cooked black beans
- ½ cup cilantro, chopped
- ½ small red onion, peeled, diced
- ½ teaspoon salt
- 1 teaspoon chipotle powder
- 2 teaspoons cumin powder
- ½ teaspoon cayenne powder
- 1 teaspoon red chili powder
- 2 tablespoons olive oil
- 8 hamburger buns, whole-wheat, toasted

Directions:

1. Prepare sweet potatoes, and for this, slice them lengthwise and roast for 40 minutes at 400 degrees F, cut-side up.
2. Prepare the burgers and for this, place all the ingredients in the bowl, except for oil and buns, stir until combined, and then shape the mixture into eight patties.
3. Take a skillet pan, place it over medium heat, add oil and when hot, add patties and cook for 4 minutes per side until browned.
4. Sandwich patties between buns, and serve.

Burrito-Stuffed Sweet Potatoes

Preparation time: 10 minutes

Cooking time: 45 minutes

Servings: 4

Ingredients:

For Sweet Potatoes:

- 1 cup cooked black beans
- 4 small sweet potatoes
- ½ cup of brown rice
- ½ teaspoon minced garlic
- 1 teaspoon tomato paste
- 1 teaspoon ground cumin
- ¼ teaspoon salt
- ½ teaspoon olive oil
- 1 ¼ cup water

For the Salsa:

- 1 cup cherry tomatoes, halved
- 1 medium red bell pepper, deseeded, chopped
- ¾ cup chopped red onion

- 2 tablespoon chopped cilantro leaves
- ½ teaspoon salt
- ¼ teaspoon ground black pepper
- 1 ½ teaspoon olive oil
- 1 tablespoon lime juice

For the Guacamole:

- 1 medium avocado, pitted, peeled
- ½ teaspoon minced garlic
- 2 tablespoons chopped cilantro leaves
- ¼ teaspoon salt
- 1 tablespoon lime juice

For Serving:

- Shredded cabbage as needed

Directions:

1. Prepare sweet potatoes and for this, place them in a baking dish, prick them with a fork and bake for 45 minutes at 400 degrees F until very tender.
2. Meanwhile, place a medium saucepan over medium heat, add rice and beans, stir in salt, oil, and tomatoes paste, pour in water and bring the mixture to boil.
3. Switch heat to medium-low level, simmer for 40 minutes until all the liquid has absorbed and set aside until

required. Prepare the salsa and for this, place all its ingredients in a bowl and stir until combined, set aside until required.
4. Prepare the guacamole and for this, place the avocado in a bowl, mash well, then add remaining ingredients, stir until combined, and set aside until required.
5. When sweet potatoes are baked, cut them along the top, pull back the skin, then split and top with rice and beans mixture.
6. Top with salsa and guacamole and cabbage and serve.

Sweet Potato, Kale and Chickpea Soup

Preparation time: 10 minutes

Cooking time: 50 minutes

Servings: 6

Ingredients:

- 3 cups cooked farro
- 3 cups chopped kale
- 1 ½ cups cooked chickpeas
- 3 cups diced sweet potatoes
- 1 red bell pepper, cored, chopped
- 1 large white onion, peeled, chopped
- ¼ teaspoon salt
- ¼ teaspoon cayenne pepper
- 2 tablespoons Thai red curry paste
- 2 tablespoons olive oil
- 2 cups of water
- 4 cups vegetable broth

Directions:

1. Take a large pot, place it over medium heat, add oil and when hot, add onion, potato and bell pepper, season with salt, and cook for 5 minutes until onions have softened.
2. Stir in curry paste, cook for 1 minute, then stir in farro, pour in water and broth, and stir until combined.
3. Bring the mixture to boil, switch heat to the low level and cook for 35 minutes.
4. Stir in kale and chickpeas, cook for 5 minutes and then stir in cayenne pepper.

Pesto with Squash Ribbons and Fettuccine

Preparation time: 10 minutes

Cooking time: 0 minute

Servings: 4

Ingredients:

For the Pesto:

- 1/3 cup pumpkin seeds, toasted
- 1 cup cilantro leaves
- 2 teaspoons chopped jalapeño, deseeded
- 1 teaspoon minced garlic
- 1 lime, juiced
- ½ teaspoon of sea salt
- ⅓ cup olive oil

For Pasta and Squash Ribbons:

- 8 ounces fettuccine, whole-grain, cooked
- 2 small zucchini
- 1 yellow squash

Directions:

1. Prepare ribbons, and for this, slice zucchini and squash by using a vegetable peeler and then set aside until required.
2. Prepare pesto, and for this, place all its ingredients in a food processor and pulse for 2 minutes until blended.
3. Place vegetable ribbons in a bowl, add cooked pasta, then add prepared pesto and toss until well coated.
4. Serve straight away.

Thai Red Curry with Vegetables

Preparation time: 10 minutes

Cooking time: 25 minutes

Servings: 4

Ingredients:

- 1 ¼ cups brown rice, cooked
- 1 cup sliced carrots
- 1 medium red bell pepper, cored, sliced into strips
- 1 green bell pepper, cored, sliced into strips
- 1 ½ cups sliced kale
- 1 teaspoon minced garlic
- 1 cup chopped white onion
- 1 tablespoon grated ginger
- 1/8 teaspoon salt
- 2 tablespoons Thai red curry paste
- 1 ½ teaspoon coconut sugar
- 1 tablespoon olive oil
- 1 tablespoon soy sauce
- 2 teaspoons lime juice
- 14 ounces of coconut milk

- ½ cup of water
- ¼ cup chopped cilantro

Directions:

1. Prepare the curry and for this, take a large skillet pan, place it over medium heat, add oil and when hot, add onion, season with salt, and cook for 5 minutes.
2. Stir in ginger and garlic, cook for 1 minute until fragrant, then add carrot and bell pepper and cook for 5 minutes.
3. Stir in curry paste, cook for 2 minutes, then add kale, stir in sugar, pour in coconut milk, stir until combined and bring the mixture to simmer.
4. Switch heat to the low level, simmer for 10 minutes until vegetables are tender, and then stir in soy sauce and lime juice.
5. Garnish with cilantro and serve with brown rice.

Thai Green Curry with Spring Vegetables

Preparation time: 10 minutes

Cooking time: 35 minutes

Servings: 4

Ingredients:

- 2 cups sliced asparagus
- 1 small white onion, peeled, diced
- 2 cups baby spinach, chopped
- 1 cup sliced carrots
- 1 teaspoon minced garlic
- 1 tablespoon chopped ginger
- 1 cup brown rice, cooked
- 2 tablespoons Thai green curry paste
- 1 ½ teaspoon coconut sugar
- 1/8 teaspoon salt
- 1 ½ teaspoon lime juice
- 2 teaspoons olive oil
- 1 ½ teaspoons soy sauce
- 14 ounces coconut milk, unsweetened

- ½ cup of water

Directions:

1. Take a large skillet pan, place it over medium heat, add oil and when hot, add ginger, onion, and garlic and cook for 5 minutes.
2. Then add carrots and asparagus, cook for 3 minutes, stir in curry paste and continue cooking for 2 minutes.
3. Pour in milk and water, stir in sugar and bring the curry to simmer.
4. Switch heat to the low level, simmer for 10 minutes until cooked, then stir in spinach and cook for 30 seconds until spinach leaves wilt.
5. When done, remove the pan from heat, stir in lime juice and soy sauce, taste to adjust seasoning and garnish with cilantro.
6. Serve curry with boiled rice.

Zucchanoush

Preparation time: 10 minutes

Cooking time: 10 minutes

Servings: 7

Ingredients:

- 1 pound small zucchini, quartered lengthwise
- 3 tablespoons mint leaves, divided
- ½ teaspoon minced garlic
- 1/3 teaspoon ground black pepper
- 2/3 teaspoon salt
- 2 tablespoons lemon juice
- 3 tablespoons olive oil, divided
- 1/4 cup tahini
- 1 tablespoon pine nuts, toasted

Directions:

1. Place zucchini pieces in a bowl, add 1 tablespoon oil, season with ½ teaspoon salt, toss until well coated, and then grill for 10 minutes over medium heat until evenly charred.

2. Then transfer grilled zucchini to a food processor, add remaining ingredients, except for mint and nuts, and process for 2 minutes until blended. Tip the mixture in a bowl, garnish with mint and nuts and then serve.

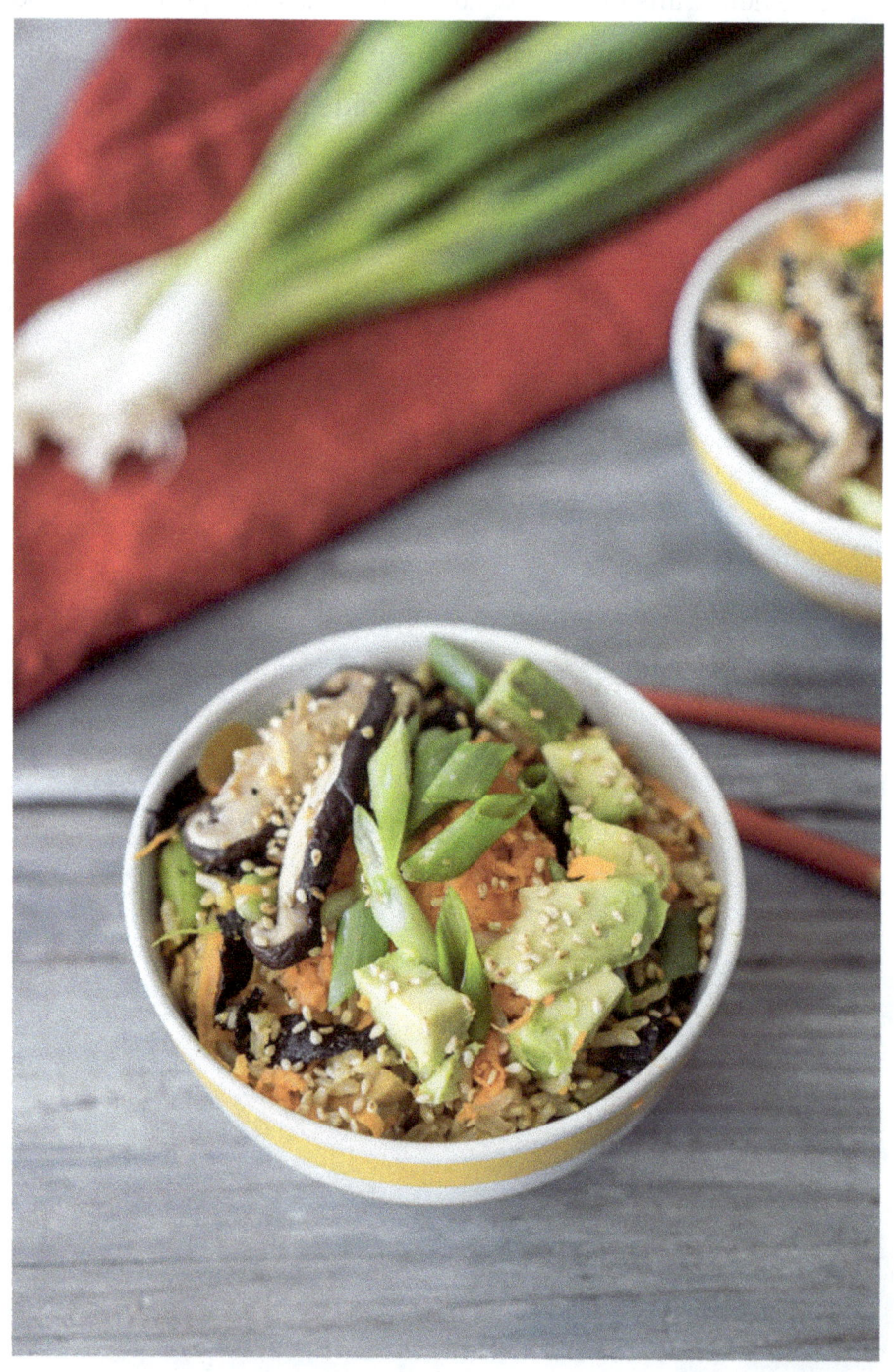

www.ingramcontent.com/pod-product-compliance
Lightning Source LLC
Chambersburg PA
CBHW070731030426
42336CB00013B/1940